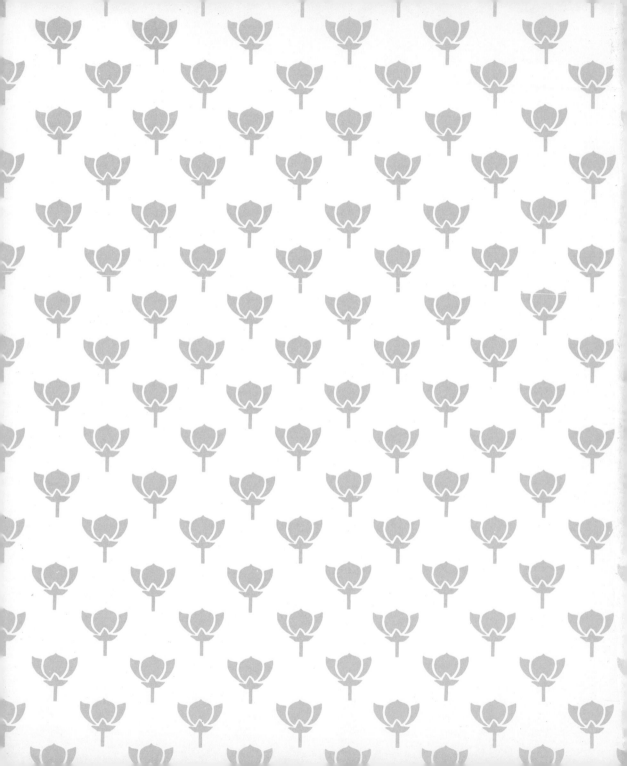

The Pregnant Woman's Journal

What's happening to me,
What's happening to my baby

by Susan and John Hopkins

Universe

Published by
Universe Books
381 Park Avenue South
© 1987 by Susan and John Hopkins
All rights reserved.
87 88 89 90 91 / 10 9 8 7 6
Printed in Hong Kong
Distributed to the trade by St. Martin's Press

The
Pregnant
Woman's
Journal

This journal is designed to promote an interest in the unique processes you will experience during your pregnancy and to stimulate a reverence for the miracle of life. It is not intended to replace your physician's care and guidance.

Every pregnancy has its own distinctive qualities, as does every baby. This information is based on average growth, development, and characteristics. Variations are common.

TO USE THIS JOURNAL:
  Turn to the NINTH MONTH. Write in your due date.
  Now work backward and forward from your due date
  filling in the remaining dates and months.

Week of _____   Week of _____

MONDAY

TUESDAY

WEDNESDAY

THURSDAY

FRIDAY

SATURDAY

SUNDAY

Weight _____   Bust _____   Waist _____   Hips _____

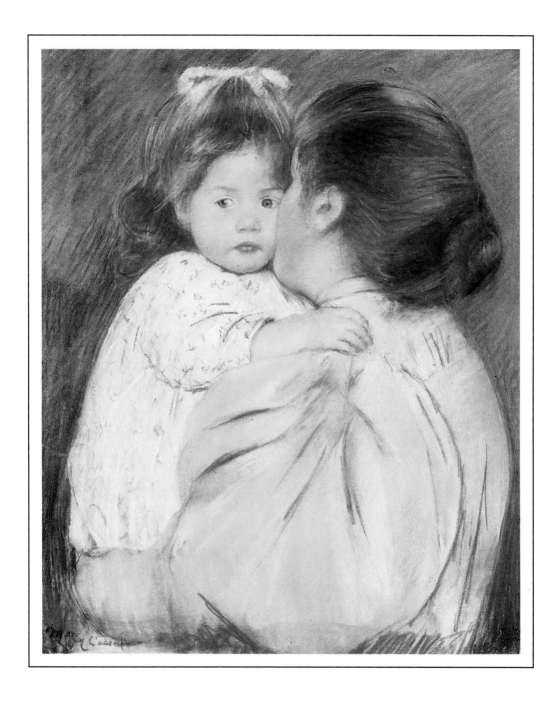

FIRST MONTH

MATERNAL DEVELOPMENT: In the first month of pregnancy most women are aware of a missed menstrual period. The breasts, in many cases, become noticeably larger and more sensitive. The nipples begin to enlarge and become broader, preparing at this early date for lactation. Four weeks after fertilization, the uterus begins to soften in consistency and assume a spherical shape, exerting slight pressure on the bladder. Nausea and vomiting, morning sickness, may be present. Fatigue is common. The uterus weighs about 2 ounces and is about 3 inches long.

FETAL DEVELOPMENT: Approximately thirty hours after fertilization, the ovum divides into two cells. Two days later a cluster of cells has developed and is floating freely in the uterus. The cluster implants itself in the wall of the uterus 6-7 days after fertilization. The woman is usually unaware of the situation since the first missed period is not due for another week. During the second week the embryo is composed of hundreds of cells which begin to form the true embryo, yolk sac, placenta, umbilical cord, and various other structures. Head folds and neural tubes develop during the third week. At the fourth week the first traces of all organs become differentiated. The heart starts beating and a primitive circulatory system exists. During this first month the embryo has increased in size 10,000 times and is now about ¼ inch long.

DUE DATES

The term of pregnancy is said to last 266 days from fertilization. Fertilization normally occurs about two weeks after the start of the last menstrual period. A common method of estimating baby's birthday is to add seven days to the date on which the last menstrual period started, then count back three months or ahead nine months. This is, of course, a tentative date. You can also count forward 40 weeks from the start of the last period. Don't become too set on your calculated date. Variations in weeks are common.

Week of _____   Week of _____

MONDAY

TUESDAY

WEDNESDAY

THURSDAY

FRIDAY

SATURDAY

SUNDAY

Weight _____   Bust _____   Waist _____   Hips _____

Week of _____ Week of _____

MONDAY

TUESDAY

WEDNESDAY

THURSDAY

FRIDAY

SATURDAY

SUNDAY

Weight _____ Bust _____ Waist _____ Hips _____

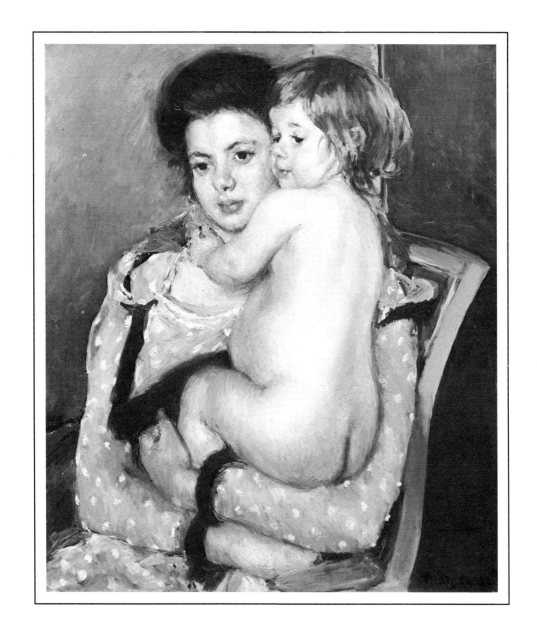

SECOND MONTH

MATERNAL DEVELOPMENT: The uterus increases in size and continues to change shape and consistency. There is more pressure on the bladder. Urinary frequency and urgency begin to increase. The breasts are becoming larger. Nausea may be more common. Fatigue increases due to metabolic changes. There may be a slight weight loss during the first two months of pregnancy. At the end of this month, the uterus is about 4 inches long.

FETAL DEVELOPMENT: The heart of the embryo is now pumping frequently but irregularly. Arms, shoulders, and hands begin to appear. The upper jaw and nose begin to form. The internal organs, nervous and circulatory systems are developing. The cartilage skeleton shows marked development as early bone cells begin to form. The stomach begins to produce digestive juices and the liver and kidneys start to function. Muscular reflexes occur but the mother has no awareness of them. Lips, tongue, and the first teeth buds appear. Due to the early development of the brain, the head is large in proportion to the rest of the body. The length of the embryo is 1 inch and the weight is 1/30 of an ounce.

NUTRITION AND DIET

Calories (per day)	2200	
Protein	65 gm.	Egg, milk, fish, meat
Calcium	1700 mg.	Milk, cheese, vegetables
Iron	18 mg.	Egg, organ meats, shellfish
Magnesium	450 mg.	Dairy products, fish, beans
Niacin	15 mg.	Milk, peanuts, organ meats
Folic Acid	0.8 mg.	Leafy vegetables, yeast
Vitamin A	6000 units	Egg, milk, vegetables
Vitamin B1	1.3 mg.	Bran, wheat germ, yeast
Vitamin B2	1.8 mg.	Liver, milk, yeast
Vitamin C	60 mg.	Citrus Fruits, vegetables
Vitamin D	400 units	Sunlight, milk, egg
Vitamin E	30 units	Vegetables, egg, butter

Week of _____ Week of _____

MONDAY

TUESDAY

WEDNESDAY

THURSDAY

FRIDAY

SATURDAY

SUNDAY

Weight _____ Bust _____ Waist _____ Hips _____

Week of _____ Week of _____

MONDAY

TUESDAY

WEDNESDAY

THURSDAY

FRIDAY

SATURDAY

SUNDAY

Weight _____ Bust _____ Waist _____ Hips _____

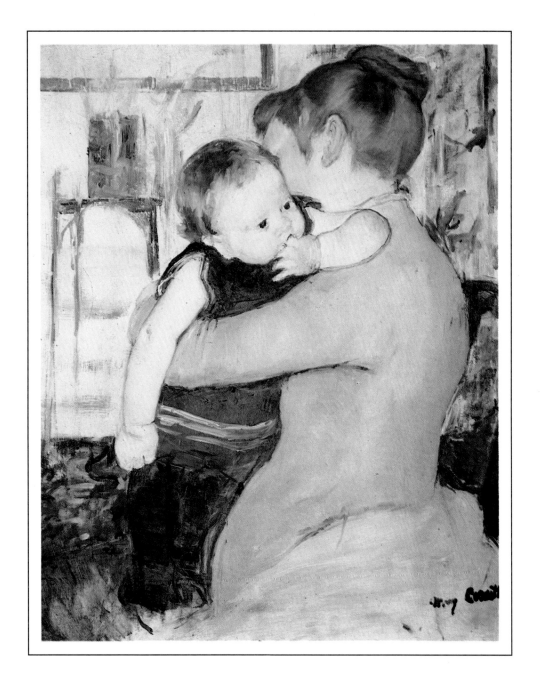

THIRD MONTH

MATERNAL DEVELOPMENT: The uterus continues to enlarge and is often the size of an orange by the twelfth post-menstrual week. It weighs about 7 ounces and contains 1-3 ounces of amniotic fluid. Pressure continues on the bladder, causing further urinary disturbance. During this month, the blood volume begins to increase, causing the heart to work harder. The pulse rate increases. Metabolic changes cause lethargy and fatigue. Colostrum, a clear fluid, may be expressed from the breasts. Weight gain is estimated at 2 pounds, though this is highly variable. This is the end of the first trimester.

FETAL DEVELOPMENT: The embryo is called the fetus after the ninth week. Rapid growth continues for all organs and systems. The sex can be determined externally. Footprints and handprints appear and remain the same for life. Nails begin to appear. The eyelids, which formed in the first month, now close for the first time. Frowning is possible. The vocal cords are formed. Swallowing of the amniotic fluid begins. Urination occurs. The thumbs move. Sperm and egg cells exist in the fetal reproductive system. In the twelfth week the fetus is about 2¾ inches long and weighs ¾ ounce.

BIBLIOGRAPHY

Bean, Constance A., *Methods of Childbirth*
Bradley, Robert A., *Husband-Coached Childbirth*
Davis, Adelle, *Let's Have Healthy Children*
Dick Read, Grantly, *Childbirth Without Fear*
De Hazell, Lester, *Commonsense Childbirth*
Flanagan, Geraldine, *The First Nine Months of Life*
Greenhill, J. P., *The Miracle of Life*
Ina May, *Spiritual Midwifery*
Ingelman-Sundberg, Axel, and Wirsen, Claes, *A Child is Born*
La Leche League International, *The Womanly Art of Breastfeeding*
Lamaze, Fernand, *Painless Childbirth-Lamaze*
Lang, Raven, *Birth Book*
Leboyer, Frederick, *Birth Without Violence*
Milinaire, Caterine, *Birth*
Olds, Sally W., and Eiger, Martin, *The Complete Book of Breastfeeding*
White, Gregory J., *Emergency Childbirth*

Week of _____   Week of _____

MONDAY

TUESDAY

WEDNESDAY

THURSDAY

FRIDAY

SATURDAY

SUNDAY

Weight _____   Bust _____   Waist _____   Hips _____

Week of _____   Week of _____

MONDAY

TUESDAY

WEDNESDAY

THURSDAY

FRIDAY

SATURDAY

SUNDAY

Weight _____ Bust _____ Waist _____ Hips _____

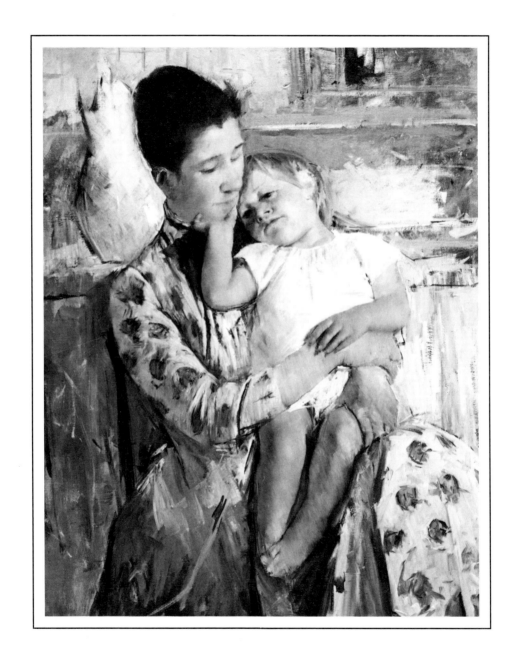

FOURTH MONTH

MATERNAL DEVELOPMENT: The uterus changes from a spherical to an ovoid shape and starts to rise from the pelvic to the abdominal cavity. Pressure on the bladder is slightly lessened. Nausea has usually disappeared by this time and the appetite increases. Fetal movements, quickening, can be felt around the sixteenth week, though they are so delicate they may go undetected for a time. Vaginal secretions may increase and are strongly acid, helping to guard against various bacterial organisms. The breasts continue to change, the nipple pigmentation perhaps darkening. The uterus weighs 18 ounces, the placenta 6 ounces. The average weight gain at this time is 8 pounds.

FETAL DEVELOPMENT: This is the beginning of the Growth Period. During the rest of the term, the fetus grows from 1 ounce to about 7¼ pounds. At this time the placenta is well developed and totally supports the fetus, supplying it with food and oxygen from the mother's blood. The umbilical cord pumps the fetal blood to and from the placenta, bringing in nutrients and removing carbon dioxide and other waste products. The two blood systems are separate and do not mingle. The fetal heart can be heard with a stethoscope and is pumping about 50 pints a day. The skeleton is visible on X-rays. Sexual organs are clearly visible. Eyelashes and eyebrows are present. Growth of hair begins. Hiccups occur. Facial features are more human and distinct. Nails begin to harden and nipples appear. Head-to-toe length is 4-6 inches and the weight is 10 ounces.

EXERCISE

Muscle tone is important during pregnancy and particularly during labor and delivery. As the pregnancy progresses, there is a forward shift in the center of balance due to the enlarging uterus. This exerts strain on the abdominal, back, and leg muscles as they must work harder to maintain body equilibrium. Daily exercise not only strengthens the muscles but promotes relaxation and a sense of well-being. Walking is especially beneficial as it conditions the muscles and stimulates the body organs. Swimming, dancing, gardening, or any other activity you participated in before conception can be helpful in keeping the body fit. Squatting, crawling, and contracting the muscles of the pelvic floor will tone the muscles most used in labor.

MONDAY

TUESDAY

WEDNESDAY

THURSDAY

FRIDAY

SATURDAY

SUNDAY

Weight _____ Bust _____ Waist _____ Hips _____

Week of _____   Week of _____

MONDAY

TUESDAY

WEDNESDAY

THURSDAY

FRIDAY

SATURDAY

SUNDAY

Weight _____   Bust _____   Waist _____   Hips _____

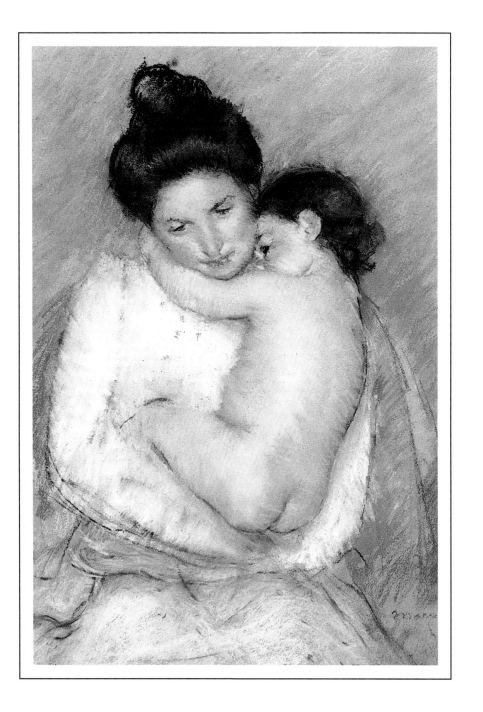

FIFTH MONTH

MATERNAL DEVELOPMENT: Halfway time. Fatigue lessens and a general sense of well-being develops. The uterus is noticeably larger and is even with the navel. Irregular, painless contractions (Braxton-Hicks contractions) can now be felt, though they have been occurring since the second month. Urinary frequency continues. Vaginal secretions may be profuse. Quickening is quite apparent now. Due to the increased blood volume and the effects of hormones, skin changes are occurring. Some women experience darkening of the skin on the forehead, nose, and cheeks. This is chloasma or "the mask of pregnancy." Many women notice tiny red blood vessels—spider angioma—on the face, neck, arms, chest, and back. All of these skin changes normally disappear within a short time of delivery. Breast growth has probably leveled off, to pick up again during the last months.

FETAL DEVELOPMENT: At this time the fetus is well developed although not very large. The head is still large in proportion to the rest of the body. The face is red and wrinkled. Fat is starting to be deposited. Lanugo—delicate, downy hair—appears on the back, arms, and legs. A whitish substance, vernix, appears on the skin. Both lanugo and vernix are often present at birth. Meconium—a fecal excretion—begins to form in the intestines. The grasp reflex is present. Fetal movements are palpable. The fetus is beginning to store iron. Enamel and dentine begin to be deposited for teeth. Head-to-toe length is 8–11 inches and the fetus weighs approximately 1¼ pounds.

RELAXATION

Relaxation exercises are extremely important to aid in the smoothness of labor and delivery. The following is one technique designed to allow you to become more conscious of your breathing and the contraction and relaxation of your muscles.
Lie on your side on a firm surface with your body supported by pillows. Begin deep sighing breathing, exhaling through an open mouth. The facial muscles, jaw, tongue, and eyelids should be heavy and relaxed. Begin with the toes and move up to the face, contracting specified muscles for short periods of time, then relaxing them. Take time with the muscles and learn how they feel when contracted and relaxed. Slow abdominal breathing should be continued throughout the relaxation session. Investigate other techniques for relaxation and make them part of your everyday routine.

Week of _____   Week of _____

MONDAY

TUESDAY

WEDNESDAY

THURSDAY

FRIDAY

SATURDAY

SUNDAY

Weight _____ Bust _____ Waist _____ Hips _____

Week of _____   Week of _____

MONDAY

TUESDAY

WEDNESDAY

THURSDAY

FRIDAY

SATURDAY

SUNDAY

Weight _____   Bust _____   Waist _____   Hips _____

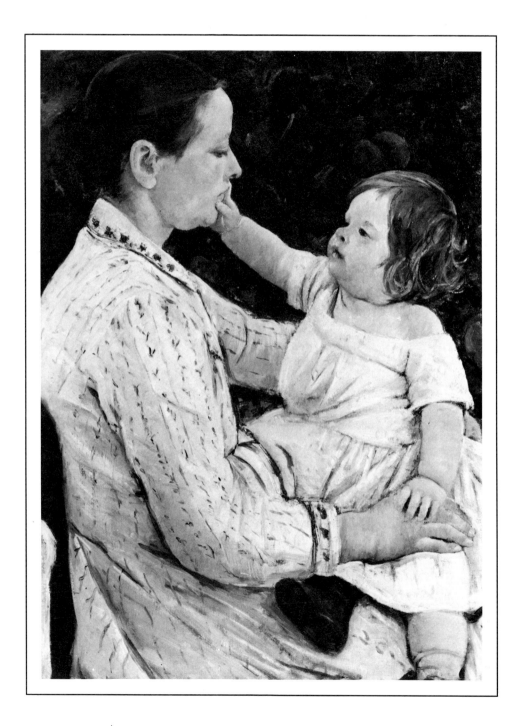

SIXTH MONTH

MATERNAL DEVELOPMENT: The uterus is slightly above the navel, causing the navel to begin to protrude. There is less pressure on the bladder. Movement and sounds of the fetus are quite evident at this time. Abdominal striae—stretch marks—may appear as the abdominal wall stretches and becomes more elastic. The linea nigra, a dark narrow line, may begin to appear mid-line from the navel to the pubis. The lining of the pelvic joints begins to soften, allowing greater mobility of the pelvis. Weight gain at this time averages 10-12 pounds, though again, this is variable.

FETAL DEVELOPMENT: The brain of the fetus is well developed although regulatory and controlling functions are not completed. The skin is red and covered with vernix. The lanugo hair begins to disappear. The umbilical cord reaches its maximum length. Thumbsucking becomes a habit. Fat is still being deposited under the skin. Fetal head-to-toe length is 11-14 inches and the weight about 2¾ pounds.

BREAST CARE

At some point, you will make the decision whether to breastfeed or bottle-feed your baby. Research the issue, talk to friends, and discuss it with your doctor. Regardless of your decision, it is important to keep your breasts in good condition. You should, by this time, be fitted with a good support brassiere, one that is adjustable and comfortable. Daily breast massage will increase circulation. To make the skin more pliable, apply a good cream or oil around the nipples and on the breasts. If you are planning to breastfeed your baby, the nipples need to be toughened in the last 6-8 weeks of pregnancy. You can gently pull the nipple, perhaps 12 times daily. You can also rub the nipples with a wet washcloth or loofah sponge while bathing. If you repeat these activities conscientiously, your breasts will be prepared and you will not likely experience discomfort in the first weeks of nursing.

CLOTHING AND EQUIPMENT

Unless you feel strongly about pink for girls and blue for boys, you might want to start thinking now about clothing and equipment for your baby. Here is a list of items that you will eventually need:

4-6 dozen diapers	baby bed
4-6 cotton shirts	3-6 crib sheets
4-6 nightgowns	waterproof sheeting
2 sweaters, front opening	bath basin
5-8 receiving blankets	2-4 bath towels
1 bunting	3 soft washcloths
1-2 knit shawls	mild soap
4-6 cotton suits	diaper pail
2 waterproof pants	safety pins
2 hats	vitamin drops

Week of _____ Week of _____

MONDAY

TUESDAY

WEDNESDAY

THURSDAY

FRIDAY

SATURDAY

SUNDAY

Weight _____ Bust _____ Waist _____ Hips _____

Week of _____   Week of _____

MONDAY

TUESDAY

WEDNESDAY

THURSDAY

FRIDAY

SATURDAY

SUNDAY

Weight _____ Bust _____ Waist _____ Hips _____

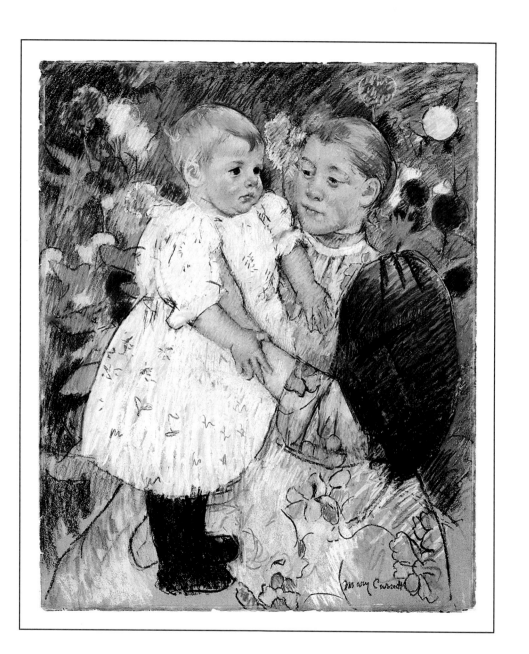

SEVENTH MONTH

MATERNAL DEVELOPMENT: The uterus is rising into the abdomen, putting pressure on the diaphragm and decreasing lung capacity. Shortness of breath occurs. The stomach is pushed up and back, sometimes causing mild indigestion. The developing uterus causes a shift in the center of gravity, sometimes resulting in poor posture and muscle cramps. The lower abdominal ligaments attached to the uterus may cramp because of the increased load they must support. Aches and pains peculiar only to the pregnant state may be experienced. The average weight gain at this time is 21 pounds. The uterus now weighs 2 pounds. Breasts have gained about 14 ounces.

FETAL DEVELOPMENT: The fetus is well developed but not yet ready for birth. Resistance to infection is low. The temperature regulation mechanism is not yet completed. The fetus is too small and weak to nurse properly. Materials such as calcium, iron, phosphorus, and nitrogen are being stored for life outside the uterus. Eyelids begin to open occasionally. Fingernails reach fingertips. The male testes begin to descend into the scrotum. Head-to-toe length is 16 inches and the fetus weighs about 3½ pounds.

PREPARED CHILDBIRTH

In the past several years there has been a trend toward natural or prepared childbirth, that is, childbirth in which both parents are active, conscious participants in the birth process. Being informed and understanding about the nature of pregnancy and birth will allow the woman and her mate to have confidence in their ability to help in the birth of their baby. There are prepared childbirth classes in many communities today. These classes ordinarily begin in the seventh month and are composed of women in the same stage of pregnancy and their mates. Besides being instructed in various exercises and the mechanics of labor and delivery, you will have the valuable opportunity to share in the feelings and experiences of others. Regardless of the eventual character of your labor and delivery, prepared childbirth classes provide an expanding life experience.

Week of _____   Week of _____

MONDAY

TUESDAY

WEDNESDAY

THURSDAY

FRIDAY

SATURDAY

SUNDAY

Weight _____ Bust _____ Waist _____ Hips _____

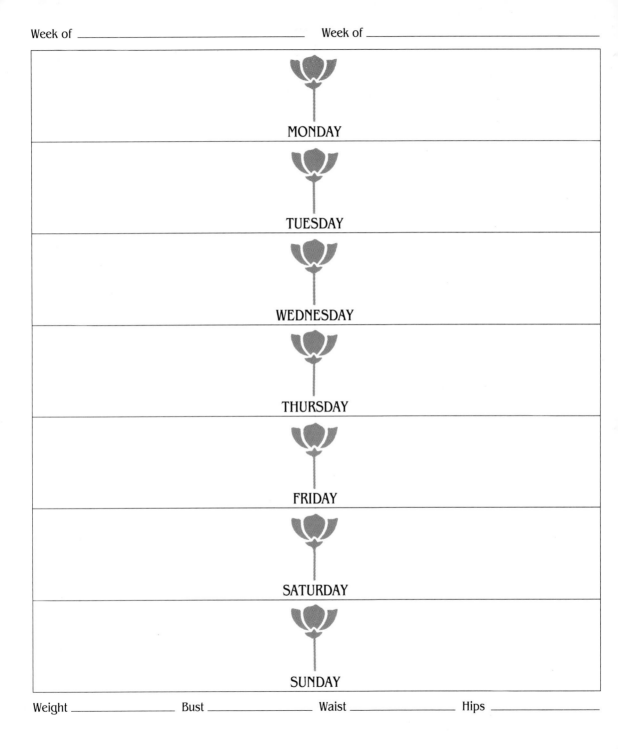

Week of _____   Week of _____

MONDAY

TUESDAY

WEDNESDAY

THURSDAY

FRIDAY

SATURDAY

SUNDAY

Weight _____ Bust _____ Waist _____ Hips _____

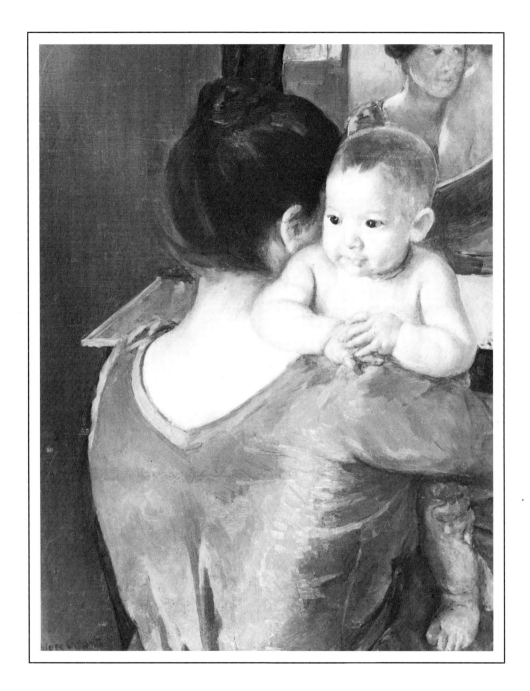

EIGHTH MONTH

MATERNAL DEVELOPMENT: The external evidence of pregnancy is notable at this time. The navel protrudes. Constipation, hemorrhoids, varicose veins, insomnia, and indigestion may occur. Leg cramps and sudden leg pains may be present due to the pressure of the fetus on nerves. Edema—swelling of the legs and ankles—may occur because of increased pressure on the blood vessels leading to the extremities. There is a large iron and calcium loss due to fetal requirements. Further softening of the pelvic joints may cause more pronounced fatigue.

FETAL DEVELOPMENT: The fetus has lost its wrinkled appearance due to fat deposits and now appears rounded and smooth. Definite wakeful periods occur. The fetus may settle into a head-down position and the earlier acrobatics lessen. Large amounts of calcium, iron, phosphorus, and nitrogen continue to be stored. Head-to-toe length is 17½ inches and the fetus weighs about 5 pounds.

BREATHING

The following breathing techniques will help you during labor. Practice daily.

Abdominal: used during the first stage of labor. Breathe in and out gently through the nostrils, mouth closed, muscles relaxed. The abdomen should rise during inhalation, drop during exhalation.

High Chest: used at the end of the first stage (transition) when the dilation is being completed and the baby begins to move through the opened cervix. Breathing is quicker. The ribs should expand laterally with each inhalation.

Push: used during the second stage when you are pushing the baby down the birth canal. Take three deep breaths through an open mouth. Hold the last breath for the duration of the contraction while pushing with the abdominal muscles. Exhale slowly and deeply at the end of each contraction.

Panting: also known as "candle blows," used at the crowning and birth of the baby's head to slow the passage through the perineal opening. Breathe rapidly and shallowly through an open, relaxed mouth.

Week of _____   Week of _____

MONDAY

TUESDAY

WEDNESDAY

THURSDAY

FRIDAY

SATURDAY

SUNDAY

Weight _____ Bust _____ Waist _____ Hips _____

Week of _____ Week of _____

MONDAY

TUESDAY

WEDNESDAY

THURSDAY

FRIDAY

SATURDAY

SUNDAY

Weight _____ Bust _____ Waist _____ Hips _____

NINTH MONTH

MATERNAL DEVELOPMENT: Full term. The uterus reaches its greatest height. Walking and sitting become more difficult. Pressure on the bladder increases and vaginal secretions increase in preparation for delivery. Braxton-Hicks contractions are more frequent and evident as the body prepares for labor. "Lightening," caused by the fetus descending into the pelvic cavity, may occur several weeks before delivery. This makes breathing easier for the woman and she may feel lighter. The fitting in, or engaging, of the fetal head may occur days or weeks before birth. As this occurs the cervix shortens and may begin to thin (efface). Some women experience a slight weight loss a few days before delivery. The average weight gain at term is $27\frac{1}{2}$ pounds. Breasts have gained about 1 pound. The uterus weighs $2\frac{1}{4}$ pounds and is 14 inches long.

FETAL DEVELOPMENT: The fetal skin is smooth and may still have lanugo about the shoulders. Vernix is present over the entire body. Nails are well developed. The scalp hair is usually dark. The eyes are slate colored, and it is impossible to detect their final color. Male testes have descended into the scrotum. Although the blood content of the fetus is only $\frac{1}{2}$ pint, the fetal heart is pumping about 600 pints a day. During these last weeks of uterine life, nitrogen, iron, and calcium are still being stored. Growth slows shortly before birth as the fetus is prepared for life outside the womb. The placenta weighs $1\frac{1}{2}$ pounds and is 7-9 inches in diameter. At term, the baby's average length is 20 inches and the average weight is $7\frac{1}{4}$ pounds.

LABOR STAGES

Each woman's labor and delivery differs. The following is a generalized explanation of the labor process.

First Stage: The dilation stage. Begins with regular uterine contractions and ends with full dilation of the cervix. This is usually the longest stage. The contractions may become progressively closer together toward the end of the stage. You may experience backache, rupture of the membranes, bloody show, excitement.

Transition: Occurs at the end of the first stage when the cervix is nearly dilated and the body is preparing for the second stage. The contractions become more intense. Confusion and irritability are common. Nausea may occur. You may experience restlessness, apprehension, frustration.

Second Stage: The expulsion stage. Begins with complete dilation of the cervix and ends with the birth of the baby. Strong spontaneous contractions of the uterus begin to move the baby down the birth canal. The pelvic floor muscles are stretched greatly as the baby's head is born. The shoulders are then born, followed by the rest of the body. You may experience relief, desire to bear down, increased energy.

Third Stage: The placental stage. The placenta first separates from the uterine wall. Then, in a series of contractions lasting from a few minutes to an hour, the placenta, membranes, and remaining fluid are expelled from the vagina. You may experience hunger, thirst, elation, exhaustion, and a sense of accomplishment.

THE POST-PARTUM PERIOD

In the hours following the birth of your baby, you are likely to feel exalted and energized, particularly if you experienced prepared childbirth and found it unnecessary to make use of the many drugs available. You must remember, at this time, that you have just been through a physically and emotionally exhausting period. Labor is exactly that—work—and it is likely the most difficult physical work your body will ever have to perform. For the first week or two following birth, the new mother is naturally in need of rest and quiet activity. Let the house go, let your mate or friends help whenever possible with the daily chores, the cooking, the errands. Many modern young mothers find it helpful to get up and about as soon as possible after birth. There is no need to immediately resume pre-birth activity, but an occasional short walk or a few simple daily exercises will help in the involution process.

Most women are concerned about weight loss and wish to return to their pre-pregnant state as quickly as possible. At birth, the average woman's weight loss is 13 pounds. It is often said that it takes approximately 6 months for a woman to regain her earlier weight status, particularly if she is nursing her child. A few weeks after the baby is born, the woman can embark on her normal physical exercise routine. The following exercises are often suggested for post-partum shape-up:

Pelvic tilt: Kneeling on all fours, arch the back, hold for a few seconds, then round the small of the back, dropping the head. Do slowly and smoothly.

Sit-ups: Lie flat on the back, with the small of the back touching the ground. Extend the hands over the head, then slowly bring the hands toward the feet, sitting up. Try to keep the feet from leaving the ground.

Abdominal: While standing or sitting, contract the abdominal muscles, hold for a few seconds, then relax.

It is important to maintain the pre-birth nutrition and diet routines you have established. If you are breastfeeding, you will need about 3,000 calories a day and are advised to step up your fluid intake, as this aids in lactation. If your baby is on a formula, you can reduce your caloric intake to 1,000 calories a day, if so advised by your physician.

Much has been said on the subject of "post-partum blues," often called "baby blues." Many women experience extreme sensitivity and depression in the weeks following childbirth; others do not. It is helpful to understand that the hormonal structure of your body has been altered greatly by the birth and it will take time before you are in balance again. If you feel like crying, cry. This is a natural release of tension and is ordinarily short-lived. Talk to your mate, your friends, and family; let out whatever feeling you are holding in check. All those concerned will then have a better understanding of the situation and can lend support and care. Most important, try to develop a long view of your situation. Keep in mind that one day soon you will fit into your pre-pregnancy wardrobe, your body will be healed, you will again be in balance, and you will be strengthened and made richer by the powerful experience of birth.

Week of _____   Week of _____

MONDAY

TUESDAY

WEDNESDAY

THURSDAY

FRIDAY

SATURDAY

SUNDAY

Weight _____   Bust _____   Waist _____   Hips _____

Week of _____   Week of _____

MONDAY

TUESDAY

WEDNESDAY

THURSDAY

FRIDAY

SATURDAY

SUNDAY

Weight _____ Bust _____ Waist _____ Hips _____

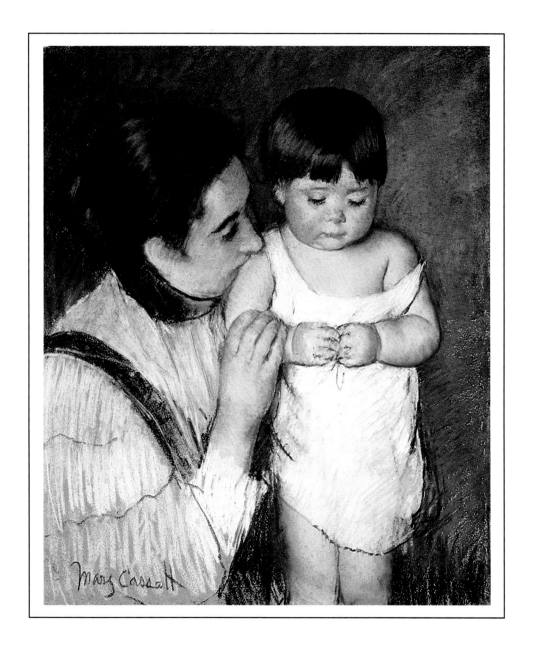

BABY'S FIRST MONTH

Following childbirth, the puerperal period begins. In this six- to eight-week period,' the woman's body undergoes decided changes. The uterus shrinks from an average 2 pounds to 3 ounces. During this time, the woman may experience uterine contractions and will have a uterine discharge, lochia, which normally lasts a few weeks. Menstruation will resume within 6-24 weeks and is likely to resume later if the mother is breastfeeding. If the new mother has had an episiotomy, she may be uncomfortable for a few days as the stitches heal. The peak of discomfort is usually the second or third day, when the swelling is most noted. One most helpful practice to ease the discomfort is to take very warm to hot sitz baths two to three times a day for 20 minutes. The heat stimulates circulation, which aids in the healing process, and also relaxes the mother. Contracting and relaxing the muscles of the pelvic floor (the Kegel exercise) will hasten the return of tone and strength to the vaginal muscles. Many women adopt the Kegel exercise into their regular physical exercise routine and continue to use it long after the birth of their babies.

*

During birth the skull bones overlap slightly to allow the baby to move more easily down the birth canal. This overlapping may cause molding of the baby's head, but this usually disappears within 24 hours. The skull parts have not yet fused so the baby's head has two noticeable fontanels, soft spots. The largest of these is on the front top of the head and gradually closes during the first 18 months of life. A few days after birth, the newborn will have his* first bowel movement, meconium, a black sticky substance. This will gradually become lighter in color until it is yellow and of grainy consistency in breastfed babies. The stools of formula-fed babies are light yellow and have a more solid consistency. The severed umbilical cord will darken, dry, and fall off within a week after birth. Newborns generally sleep 12–16 hours a day. They have the ability to see, hear, suck, cry, yawn, stretch, digest milk, and eliminate wastes. The eyes react to light but cannot focus for a few weeks. The hands are usually clenched.

*The universal pronoun "he" is used when referring to the baby. This is done solely for convenience and is meant to indicate male and female.

Week of _____ Week of _____

MONDAY

TUESDAY

WEDNESDAY

THURSDAY

FRIDAY

SATURDAY

SUNDAY

Weight _____ Bust _____ Waist _____ Hips _____

Week of _____ Week of _____

MONDAY

TUESDAY

WEDNESDAY

THURSDAY

FRIDAY

SATURDAY

SUNDAY

Weight _____ Bust _____ Waist _____ Hips _____

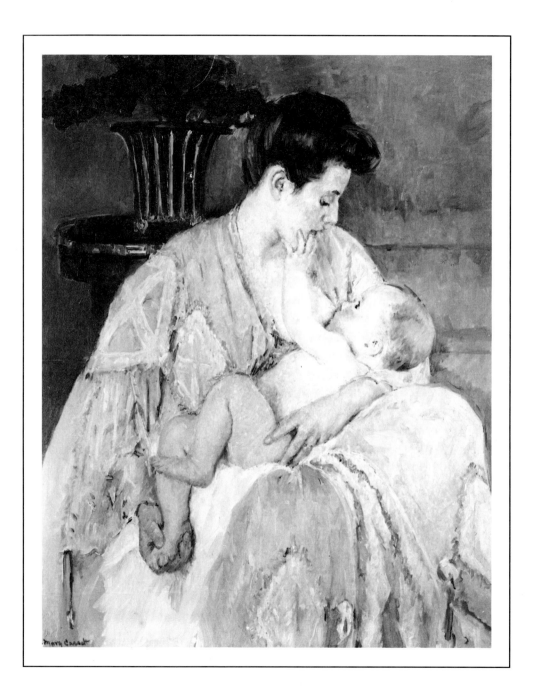

BABY'S SECOND MONTH

The baby's muscles are beginning to acquire tone. He is able to lift his head briefly and turn it from side to side while lying on his abdomen. The eyes focus and the baby will stare at lights, windows, and large objects. He will begin to follow moving objects with his eyes. His weight gain at this time is approximately 2 pounds. Some babies of this age sleep 14-18 hours a day, others sleep much less. The baby will smile in response to a friendly touch and loving voice. He will begin to utter a variety of sounds. These throaty vocalizations are the beginnings of speech. You can encourage him by repeating these basic sounds, talking to him in normal tones, making funny sounds, and singing to him. The baby begins by grasping the world with his eyes. A colorful, interesting environment will encourage his curiosity.

These first reflexes are present in the first few months:

Sucking: When the baby's mouth is touched, eager sucking motions are made.

Moro: The startle reflex. A rapid change in position or sudden noise causes the baby to suddenly fling his arms outward with the hands open.

Grasp: Stimulation of the palms and soles of the feet leads to a closing and gripping of the hands and a curling of the toes.

Rooting: Touching of the baby's cheek elicits head turning in that direction.

NUTRITION AND DIET

For the first 24 hours after birth the baby's digestive system does nothing except empty itself of meconium. During this time bacteria enters the system and the baby is ready to digest food. Colostrum is ideal at this time because of its high protein and low fat content. For the first 4-5 months, the baby receives all the nutrients he needs from breast milk or a very good formula. Many doctors also recommend vitamin drops during this period. The emotional and physiological needs of the baby can be met by feeding him promptly when he cries for it and feeding him all he wants at every feeding. Until around the sixth week of life, the baby can only suck. Sucking helps develop the lower jaw, so allowing the baby's sucking needs to be fulfilled. From the eight to the twelfth week the baby learns to mouth and swallow strained foods. Around the twelfth week the baby will enjoy the introduction of strained vegetables and fruits. These should be introduced gradually, one at a time, the same food for a 4-5 day period. Meats, egg yolk, and liver can be introduced around 5-6 months. In the third month many babies like to chew on objects to help begin the process of teething. Raw carrots cooled in the refrigerator or commercial teethers are helpful at this time.

Week of _____   Week of _____

MONDAY

TUESDAY

WEDNESDAY

THURSDAY

FRIDAY

SATURDAY

SUNDAY

Weight _____   Bust _____   Waist _____   Hips _____

Week of _____   Week of _____

MONDAY

TUESDAY

WEDNESDAY

THURSDAY

FRIDAY

SATURDAY

SUNDAY

Weight _____   Bust _____   Waist _____   Hips _____

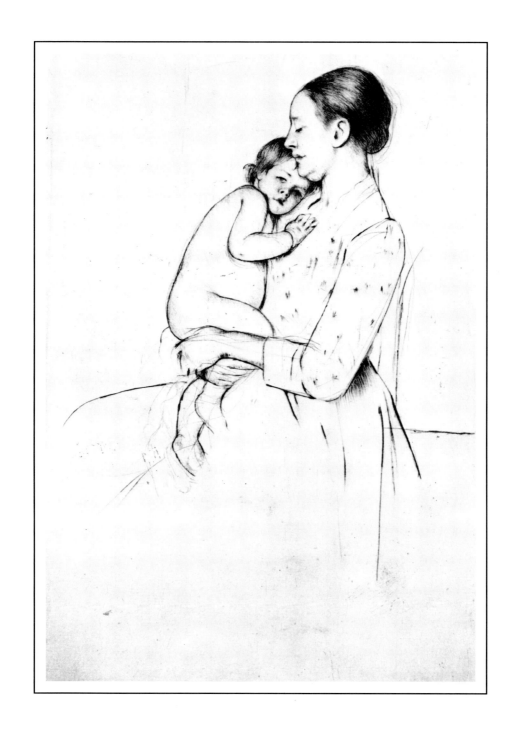

BABY'S THIRD MONTH

The baby is gaining more control of his head and is able to bear weight on his forearms. During the third month the Babinski reflex appears: When the sole of the foot is stroked, the toes turn upward and spread outward. This reflex will last until the child is about 2 years old. The baby will soon notice his hands and will enjoy watching them move in front of his face. The hands are no longer continuously fisted; the fingers are open and in motion. The baby is becoming more vocal, chuckling, cooing, gurgling, and developing a varied repertoire of sounds. He is responsive to objects and people and becomes still at times when he hears conversation or an unfamiliar sound. He may give up his late night feeding at this time, though many babies continue to need this feeding for another month. The baby has gained about 2 pounds per month, or 6 pounds. The average baby of this age sleeps 12-16 hours a day.

BONDING

This is a time of immense joy for both parent and child as well as being an important bonding period. The baby responds readily to his environment and expresses pleasure at feeding, bathing, being held and snuggled. He is, at this young age, developing the capacity for love, trust, tenderness, and compassion by having his physical and psychological needs met promptly with care and patience. You can help your baby build a solid emotional base by being generous with yourself and respecting him as an individual human being. Enjoy your child. Hold him, kiss him, talk and sing to him as much as you like. You will supply him with an optimistic, delightful view of the world. By giving of yourself, you will experience personal growth and expansion and will be blessed with a happy, generous child.

BIBLIOGRAPHY

Dodson, Fitzhugh, *How to Parent*
Gesell, Arnold, and Ilg, Francis. *Infant and Child in the Culture of Today*
Glover, Leland, *How to Give Your Child a Good Start in Life*
Greenberg, Sidonie, *The New Encyclopedia of Child Care and Guidance*
Newton, Niles, *The Family Book of Child Care*
Spock, Benjamin, *Baby and Child Care*

Week of _____   Week of _____

MONDAY

TUESDAY

WEDNESDAY

THURSDAY

FRIDAY

SATURDAY

SUNDAY

Weight _____   Bust _____   Waist _____   Hips _____

Week of _____ Week of _____

MONDAY

TUESDAY

WEDNESDAY

THURSDAY

FRIDAY

SATURDAY

SUNDAY

Weight _____ Bust _____ Waist _____ Hips _____

Week of _____   Week of _____

MONDAY

TUESDAY

WEDNESDAY

THURSDAY

FRIDAY

SATURDAY

SUNDAY

Weight _____   Bust _____   Waist _____   Hips _____

BABY'S GIFTS

From _____

Description _____

_____

_____

From _____

Description _____

_____

_____

From _____

Description _____

_____

_____

From _____

Description _____

_____

_____

From _____

Description _____

_____

_____

From _____

Description _____

_____

_____

From _____

Description _____

_____

_____

From _____

Description _____

_____

_____

From _____

Description _____

_____

_____

From _____

Description _____

_____

_____

IMPORTANT NUMBERS

Ambulance _____   Fire Department _____

_____   _____

Baby Sitter _____   General Practitioner _____

_____   _____

Childbirth Center _____   Gynecologist _____

_____   _____

Cleaner _____   Hospital _____

_____   _____

Dentist _____   Obstetrician _____

_____   _____

Diaper Service _____   Pediatrician _____

_____   _____

Druggist _____   Police Department _____

_____   _____

Emergency _____   Taxicab _____

_____   _____

_____   _____

_____   _____

All works are by the American artist Mary Cassatt (1844–1926)

1st month: *Mother and Child (Maternal Kiss),* pastel 22″ × 18″.
   Philadelphia Museum of Art, bequest of Anne Hinchman
2d month: *Reine Lefebure Holding a Nude Baby;* oil on canvas, 26¹³⁄₁₆
   ″ × 22⁹⁄₁₆″. Worcester Art Museum
3d month: *Mother and Child,* c. 1889; oil on canvas 29″ × 23½″.
   The Cincinnati Art Museum, John J. Emery Endowment
4th month: *Mother and Child* (detail), c. 1890; oil on canvas, 35⅜″ × 25⅜″.
   Courtesy of the Wichita Art Museum, The Roland P. Murdock
   Collection
5th month: *Mother and Child,* 1880; pastel on paper, 33⁷⁄₁₆″ × 29″.
   Courtesy of the Art Institute of Chicago
6th month: *The Child's Caress,* c. 1891; oil on canvas, 25½″ × 19⅝″.
   Honolulu Academy of Arts, gift in memory of Wilhelmina Tenny, 1953
7th month: *In the Garden;* pastel, 28¾″ × 23⅝″. The Baltimore Museum
   of Art, The Cone Collection, formed by Dr. Clairbel Cone and Miss Etta Cone of Baltimore, Maryland
8th month: *Mother and Child,* 1900; oil on canvas, 27⅛″ × 20⅜″. The
   Brooklyn Museum, Carl H. De Silver Fund
Baby's first month: *Young Thomas and His Mother;* colored chalks on
   board, 24″ × 20″. Pennsylvania Academy of Fine Arts, gift of Mrs. Clement Newbold
Baby's 2d month: *Mother and Child,* c. 1900; oil on canvas, 39⅝″ × 32⅛″.
   Courtesy of The Art Institute of Chicago, gift of Alexander Stewart
Baby's third month: *Quietude,* 1891; drypoint, 10⅛″ × 6¼″. The Baltimore
   Museum of Art, George A. Lucas Collection, on indefinite loan from The
   Maryland Institute

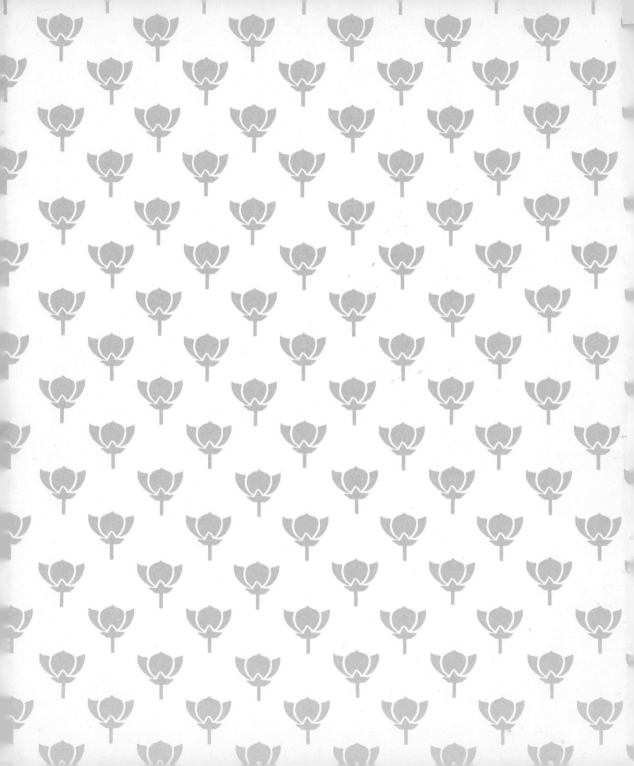